TENSION HEADACHE DIET FOR NEWLY DIAGNOSED

Discover Effective Techniques, Meal Plans, Proven Strategies, Nutritional Insights, And Self-Care Practices To Alleviate Pain And Enhance Well-Being

DR. ERIC TRISTAN

CONTENTS

CHAPTER ONE..10

Introduction 10

Comprehension Of Tension Headaches..........10

Dietary Influence On Tension Headaches.......11

Stress And Hydration-Related Headaches 13

Coffee And Its Consequences.......................14

Tension Headache Diet: Nutritional Selections To Alleviate Pain.......................................16

CHAPTER TWO..18

Food Triggers To Avoid: Uncovering The Culprits Behind Tension Headaches 18

Natural Headache Relief Through The Ingestion Of Magnesium-Rich Foods 20

The Potential Of Vitamin B2 (Riboflavin) In The Diet To Prevent Headaches...........................21

Headache Relief Via Omega-3 Fatty Acids And Anti-Inflammatory Foods: Balancing Inflammation..23

CHAPTER THREE 26

Regular And Well-Balanced Meals To Alleviate Tension Headaches....................................26

The Significance Of Sufficient Sleep In The Management Of Tension Headaches 28

Practices Of Mindful Eating To Alleviate Tension Headaches............29

Herbal Remedies And Teas For The Relief Of Tension Headaches............30

Potential Food Sensitivities And Allergies In Tension Headaches............31

CHAPTER FOUR............34

Alcohol And Tension Headaches: A Moderate Approach To Balance............34

Limiting Processed Foods: A Critical Component In The Management Of Tension Headaches ...35

A Holistic Approach To Meal Planning For Tension Headache Prevention 37

Engaging In Consultations With Healthcare Professionals: The Significance Of Expert Opinion 39

Conclusion............42

THE END 44

DISCLAIMER

The information provided in this book, is intended for informational purposes only. The content is not intended to be a substitute for professional medical advice, diagnosis, or treatment. Always seek the advice of your physician or other qualified health provider with any questions you may have regarding a medical condition. Never disregard professional medical advice or delay in seeking it because of something you have read in this book.

The author of this book has made reasonable efforts to ensure that the information provided is accurate and up-to-date at the time of publication. However, the author makes no representations or warranties of any kind, express or implied, about the completeness, accuracy, reliability, suitability, or availability of the information contained within these pages.

Any reliance you place on the information provided in this book is strictly at your own risk. The author shall not be liable for any loss, injury, or damage arising from the use of this book or the information contained herein.

The mention or reference to any individuals, products, websites, organizations, or other names within this book does not imply endorsement by the author. The inclusion of such references is solely for informational purposes and does not constitute an endorsement or recommendation.

Furthermore, the author disclaims any association or affiliation with any individuals, products, websites, organizations, or other names mentioned in this book.

It is important to consult with a qualified healthcare professional before making any dietary or lifestyle changes, especially if you have a medical condition. Each individual's health situation is unique, and what works for one person may not work for another.

Again, the information provided in this book is not intended to diagnose, treat, cure, or prevent any disease or health condition. Always seek the advice of a physician or other qualified health provider regarding any medical questions or concerns you may have.

Thank you for your understanding and for taking the necessary precautions when considering the information presented in this book.

<u>ABOUT THIS BOOK</u>

This "Tension Headache Diet" is an all-encompassing and indispensable manual that assists users in identifying and implementing dietary interventions that effectively prevent and manage tension headaches.

An extensive "Introduction" provides context for comprehending the intricacies of tension migraines and their consequences in everyday existence. Following this, the reader is provided with an in-depth analysis of "Understanding Tension Headaches," which examines the multitude of factors that contribute to this prevalent condition.

A critical element of this book is its examination of the "Role of Diet in Tension Headaches," which underscores the significant impact that dietary decisions can exert on the frequency and intensity of headaches. The chapters devoted to "Hydration and Tension Headaches" and "Caffeine and its Impact" offer significant perspectives on frequently disregarded elements that contribute to headaches. The incorporation of "Trigger Foods to Avoid" provides pragmatic recommendations for avoiding potential sources of headaches.

This book adopts a comprehensive viewpoint by examining nutritional components that may have a beneficial effect on tension headaches, including "Omega-3 Fatty Acids and Anti-Inflammatory Foods," "Incorporating Magnesium-Rich Foods," and "Vitamin B2 (Riboflavin) in the Diet." It emphasizes the value of a well-rounded approach and explores the significance of "Balanced and Regular Meals" and "Adequate Sleep" in the prevention of headaches.

This book not only addresses dietary considerations but also proposes "Mindful Eating Practices" and investigates the potential advantages of "Herbal Teas and Remedies." The section titled "Potential Food Allergies and Sensitivities" examines the relationship between food and allergies or sensitivities, and emphasizes the influence of processed foods and alcohol on tension headaches.

This book incorporates practical advice by incorporating the section titled "Meal Planning for Tension Headache Prevention," which presents readers with tangible measures to implement the suggested dietary modifications into their everyday schedules. In "Consulting with a Healthcare Professional," the book concludes with a vital reminder to seek professional guidance. This emphasizes the significance of adopting a personalized and well-informed approach to the management of tension headaches. In general, "Tension Headache Diet" serves as a fundamental resource, providing readers with the knowledge and ability to select nutritious foods that mitigate and prevent tension headaches, thereby promoting enhanced general health.

CHAPTER ONE

Introduction

Tension headaches are a widely prevalent type of headache that affects individuals on a global scale. Headaches that are mild to moderate in intensity and persistent in nature, these headaches are frequently induced by external factors such as muscle tension, stress, or muscle tension. Although there are numerous treatment options available, such as medication and lifestyle modifications, the function of diet in the management of tension migraines merits particular consideration. A comprehensive understanding of the potential effects of particular dietary selections on tension migraines is essential for those in search of natural and holistic methods to alleviate these discomforting conditions.

Comprehension Of Tension Headaches

Before exploring the correlation between diet and tension headaches, it is crucial to have a comprehensive understanding of the nature of tension headaches. Tension headaches, in contrast to migraines, do not commonly manifest symptoms such as vertigo, vomiting, or sensitivity to light and sound. Conversely, they frequently manifest as sluggish, persistent headaches that may spread to both cranial sides. In addition to stress and muscle tension, emotional strain, sleep deprivation, and inadequate posture are additional contributory elements in the pathogenesis of tension headaches.

To manage tension migraines, both the underlying causes and immediate symptoms must be addressed. Although medication may offer some degree of alleviation, a more holistic strategy encompassing adjustments to one's lifestyle, stress management strategies, and dietary regimen can prove advantageous.

Dietary Influence On Tension Headaches

Considering the importance of diet to overall health, its influence on tension migraines is becoming increasingly apparent. Specific food items and beverages may alleviate tension migraines or exacerbate their symptoms. To adopt a diet that is conducive to tension headaches, one must identify trigger foods and replace them with alternatives that may provide some symptom relief.

It is critical to completely avoid potential stimuli. Common trigger foods include nitrate-containing processed meats, aged cheese, chocolate, and foods that contain excessive amounts of additives or preservatives. Furthermore, headache-inducing blood sugar fluctuations can be avoided by adhering to a regular consumption schedule and avoiding meal missing.

However, it can be advantageous to include foods that are abundant in magnesium in one's dietary regimen. A mineral implicated in muscle relaxation and function, magnesium has been associated with the prevention of headaches. Magnesium is abundant in foods including whole cereals, legumes, leafy green vegetables, and seeds.

Stress And Hydration-Related Headaches

Dehydration frequently induces tension-related migraines. Low fluid consumption can result in reduced blood volume, which can have detrimental effects on blood flow to the brain and give rise to migraines. Hence, ensuring adequate hydration is a straightforward yet efficacious method to prevent and manage tension migraines.

To maintain proper hydration, water is the optimal beverage; individuals should strive to ingest a sufficient quantity throughout the day. Caffeinated and sugary beverages may promote dehydration; therefore, they should be consumed in moderation. Urine color is a useful indicator of hydration; urine that is light yellow to clear in color indicates adequate fluid consumption.

It is advantageous to include hydrating dishes in one's diet, in addition to water. Water-dense fruits and vegetables, including citrus, cucumber, and watermelon, can aid in maintaining adequate hydration levels. By incorporating these foods into one's diet, headache prevention can be supported deliciously and effectively.

Coffee And Its Consequences

Caffeine, which is present in specific medications, coffee, tea, and chocolate, among other natural stimulants, can exert both beneficial and detrimental impacts on tension migraines. Although caffeine may offer transient alleviation through vasoconstriction and analgesia, abrupt or excessive cessation may result in residual migraines.

Regarding caffeine consumption, moderation is vital. Individuals who are susceptible to tension migraines should maintain a steady caffeine consumption pattern as opposed to abruptly ceasing or substantially increasing their intake. Additionally, it is crucial to exercise caution regarding concealed sources of caffeine, including specific medications and energy beverages.

Withdrawal headaches from caffeine can be avoided in certain circumstances by reducing consumption progressively as opposed to ceasing abruptly. Furthermore, individuals must recognize and accommodate their personal caffeine sensitivity when it comes to caffeine intake. Maintaining a headache journal that encompasses caffeine consumption can facilitate the identification of recurring trends and inform modifications aimed at enhancing headache management.

In conclusion, achieving a diet that is conducive to tension headaches requires a multifaceted approach that encompasses eliminating trigger foods, maintaining adequate hydration, and controlling caffeine consumption. Although dietary modifications may not completely eradicate tension migraines, they can substantially mitigate the frequency and intensity of such episodes. When confronted with health-related issues, individuals should seek personalized advice and guidance from healthcare professionals by their particular circumstances and requirements.

Tension Headache Diet: Nutritional Selections To Alleviate Pain

Tension migraines, which are distinguished by a dull, persistent pain that frequently encircles the skull, have the potential to greatly impair an individual's quality of life.

Although tension migraines are caused by a variety of factors (stress, muscle tension, poor posture, etc.), dietary selections have a significant impact on whether they exacerbate or alleviate this prevalent condition.

Managing trigger foods, implementing magnesium-rich foods, ensuring adequate Vitamin B2 (riboflavin) intake, and imbibing Omega-3 fatty acids and anti-inflammatory foods are all components of a tension headache-friendly diet.

CHAPTER TWO

Food Triggers To Avoid: Uncovering The Culprits Behind Tension Headaches

Specific dietary items and beverages have been recognized as possible inciters of tension-related migraines. Although stimuli can differ among individuals, the following are some prevalent culprits:

1. Although caffeine may offer transient alleviation for headaches, sudden cessation or excessive intake may result in the development of rebound headaches. It is critical to remain hydrated and maintain a consistent caffeine intake.

2. Alcohol: Specific alcoholic beverages, including red wine, beer, and spirits, comprise chemical constituents that have the potential to induce migraines in susceptible individuals. Water retention and moderation are both essential for mitigating the effects.

3. Caffeine and additional compounds that induce headaches are present in chocolate, rendering it a possible trigger. It is advisable for those who are susceptible to tension migraines to reduce their consumption of chocolate.

4. Processed foods, which frequently contain additives such as artificial sweeteners and monosodium glutamate (MSG), have been associated with migraines in certain individuals. Choosing unadulterated, whole foods can be advantageous.

5. Aged cheeses, including blue and cheddar, contain tyramine, a compound associated with migraines. By restricting their consumption, these cheeses may contribute to a decrease in the frequency of tension migraines.

6. Nitrate-rich Foods: Certain individuals may experience migraines when consuming nitrate-rich foods, including processed meats—such as bacon and hot dogs. As an alternative, one might consider

incorporating lean proteins and selecting options that are free from nitrates.

Natural Headache Relief Through The Ingestion Of Magnesium-Rich Foods

Magnesium is an essential mineral that facilitates nerve transmission and muscle function. According to research, a magnesium deficiency might increase the frequency and severity of tension migraines. Magnesium-rich foods can be incorporated into the diet as a natural and effective remedy for these headaches:

1. Magnesium is found in abundance in spinach, kale, and Swiss chard, among other leafy greens. By integrating these leafy greens into salads, and smoothies, or serving them as side dishes, one can enhance their magnesium intake.

2. Nuts and Seeds: In addition to being delicious treats, almonds, cashews, pumpkin seeds, and sunflower seeds are also excellent sources of magnesium. Including a scattering of almonds or

seeds in one's daily diet has the potential to enhance magnesium levels.

3. Whole cereals, including quinoa, barley, and brown rice, are rich in magnesium and other vital nutrients. Selecting whole grain alternatives rather than refined cereals is a nutritious dietary decision that can aid in the management of tension migraines.

4. Magnesium-rich legumes, including chickpeas, lentils, and beans, can be incorporated into a variety of dishes, including soups, stews, and salads.

5. Fish: In addition to omega-3 fatty acids, fatty fish such as mackerel and salmon contribute to magnesium consumption. Fish consumption a few times per week may be advantageous for individuals who suffer from tension headaches.

The Potential Of Vitamin B2 (Riboflavin) In The Diet To Prevent Headaches

Vitamin B2, alternatively referred to as riboflavin, is an essential water-soluble vitamin that is critical for the maintenance of healthy skin, eyes, and neuronal function, as well as the production of energy. Some research indicates that supplementation with riboflavin may aid in the prevention of tension headaches and migraines. To incorporate this vitamin into your diet naturally:

1. Dairy products, including cheese, yogurt, and milk, are rich in riboflavin. Choose non-fat or low-fat dairy alternatives to improve your health.

2. Lean Meats: Riboflavin is present in lean portions of beef, poultry, and turkey. Opting for lean protein sources aids in the management of overall health and potentially aids in the prevention of headaches.

3. Particularly the center of an egg is rich in riboflavin. Incorporating eggs into one's dietary regimen offers a multipurpose and nourishing provision of this vital nutrient.

4. In addition to being high in magnesium, green leafy vegetables such as spinach, broccoli, and asparagus also contain riboflavin. A variety of

vegetables incorporated into one's diet is beneficial to overall health.

5. Nuts and Seeds Nuts and seeds also provide riboflavin, in addition to magnesium. Including seeds in your diet or snacking on a fistful of almonds provides an additional nutrient boost.

Headache Relief Via Omega-3 Fatty Acids And Anti-Inflammatory Foods: Balancing Inflammation

It is hypothesized that chronic inflammation plays a role in the pathogenesis and maintenance of tension migraines. With their well-documented anti-inflammatory characteristics, omega-3 fatty acids may play a pivotal role in inflammation management and the promotion of general health:

1. Sardines, mackerel, and salmon are all excellent sources of omega-3 fatty acids. Consistent ingestion of fatty fish may aid in the mitigation of inflammation and promote cognitive well-being.

2. Flaxseeds and chia seeds are exceptional sources of omega-3 fatty acids derived from plants. Simply incorporating them into smoothies, sprinkling them on yogurt, or baking products are all practical methods of increasing one's omega-3 consumption.

3. Walnuts distinguish themselves among seeds by their substantial concentration of omega-3 fatty acids. Incorporating walnuts into salads, oatmeal, or snacks can be a delicious way to incorporate them into your diet.

4. Berries: In addition to being abundant in antioxidants, blueberries, strawberries, and raspberries also possess anti-inflammatory properties. A diversity of berries consumed daily may aid in the prevention of headaches.

5. Leafy Greens: Omega-3 fatty acids are found in leafy greens such as kale and spinach, in addition to magnesium and riboflavin. These greens are multipurpose and can be integrated into prepared dishes, smoothies, and salads.

In summary, the implementation of a tension headache-friendly diet necessitates a comprehensive strategy that takes into account the exclusion of trigger foods, the consumption of foods rich in magnesium, the provision of sufficient Vitamin B2 intake, the adoption of omega-3 fatty acids and anti-inflammatory foods. Although personal reactions to dietary modifications may differ, exercising discernment and purpose in decision-making can positively impact the management of headaches and overall health. For personalized guidance and to definitively rule out any underlying medical conditions, it is recommended to seek the advice of a healthcare professional.

CHAPTER THREE

Regular And Well-Balanced Meals To Alleviate Tension Headaches

Maintaining a regular and well-balanced meal routine is an essential component in effectively managing tension migraines, which can be incited or worsened by a multitude of factors. The relationship between diet and migraines is complex, and the adoption of nutritious eating practices can substantially aid in the mitigation of tension headache frequency and intensity.

To effectively manage tension headaches, it is critical to incorporate a variety of nutritious lipids, carbohydrates, and proteins into well-balanced meals. Illnesses in the susceptibility of individuals to migraines may result from fluctuations in blood sugar levels caused by irregular eating patterns, meal avoidance, or unbalanced diets. To establish a consistent and nourishing eating regimen, it is recommended that individuals strive for three primary meals daily, with the possibility of supplementing with nutritious munchies when necessary.

The consumption of fruits, vegetables, and whole cereals, which are all complex carbohydrates, can assist in the stabilization of blood sugar levels. These foods promote a gradual release of energy, which inhibits abrupt fluctuations in blood glucose levels that could potentially contribute to migraines. Furthermore, the incorporation of lean proteins and healthy lipids into every meal serves to enhance satiety and maintain energy levels over the course of the day.

Ensuring adherence to a regular meal schedule is of equal significance. The body's circadian rhythm may be perturbed by irregular dietary patterns, which may result in tension migraines. By implementing a consistent mealtime schedule, individuals can effectively manage their blood sugar and hormone levels, thereby enhancing their ability to prevent headaches.

The Significance Of Sufficient Sleep In The Management Of Tension Headaches

Sufficient and high-quality sleep is an essential element of holistic well-being, and its influence on the management of tension headaches should not be underestimated. Insomnia and diminished sleep quality are substantial risk factors for the development and worsening of tension migraines.

Sleep hygiene, also known as establishing a regular sleep regimen, is of the utmost importance for strain headache sufferers.

Establishing regular wake-up and bedtimes assists in the regulation of the body's circadian rhythm, thereby facilitating a more anticipated sleep cycle. Implementing a soothing pre-sleep regimen, such as engaging in a heated bath or reading, can effectively communicate to the body that it is time to unwind, thereby increasing the probability of experiencing a restorative slumber.

It is crucial to consider potential sleep disorders, including sleep apnea and insomnia when it comes to managing tension headaches. Seeking guidance from a healthcare professional for the diagnosis and treatment of latent sleep disorders can result in substantial reductions in both the frequency and intensity of headaches.

Practices Of Mindful Eating To Alleviate Tension Headaches

Practicing mindful dining entails directing one's complete focus toward the sensory encounter of food, encompassing its flavor, consistency, and fragrance. Engaging in this activity may prove especially advantageous for those who are afflicted with tension migraines, given that it promotes an increased consciousness regarding dietary patterns and possible triggers.

By doing so, one can incorporate mindfulness into their meals by relishing each mouthful, decelerating the eating process, and remaining completely present throughout. By avoiding electronic device perusing and television viewing, individuals can concentrate on their cuisine and the emotions it evokes.

Mindful dining encompasses the ability to identify signals of hunger and satiety. By consuming food only when one feels truly famished and ceasing consumption when one is comfortably full, tension migraines can be avoided, which are frequently induced by overeating. A further benefit of being attuned to emotional signals associated with food is the ability to recognize and resolve stress-induced eating, which may be a factor in tension headaches.

Herbal Remedies And Teas For The Relief Of Tension Headaches

For centuries, herbal remedies and teas have been employed to mitigate a wide range of afflictions, including migraines. Along with other lifestyle adjustments, the inclusion of specific botanicals in one's diet may provide natural alleviation for tension migraines.

For instance, the muscle-relaxing properties of peppermint tea may assist in alleviating tension in the head and neck. The calming and anti-inflammatory properties of chamomile tea may provide respite from headaches caused by tension. Due to its anti-inflammatory and anti-nausea properties, ginger tea may also be useful for relieving tension migraines.

In addition to infusions, feverfew, and butterbur have demonstrated potential as herbal remedies for mitigating the frequency and severity of tension headaches. Before incorporating new botanicals or supplements into the diet, it is essential to consult a healthcare professional, as they may interact with medications or be contraindicated for specific health conditions.

Potential Food Sensitivities And Allergies In Tension Headaches

Certain individuals may experience tension migraines due to food or ingredient triggers that provoke an allergy or sensitivity. It can be critical to identify and eliminate potential triggers of tension headaches to effectively manage and prevent them.

Specific food preservatives, additives, and artificial sweeteners frequently provoke migraines. Tyramine, an additional potential trigger, is a compound that is present in matured cheeses, processed meats, and specific fermented foods. Maintaining an elaborate food journal can assist individuals in identifying particular foods that occur concurrently with episodes of headaches, thereby facilitating the detection of potential triggers.

When identifying triggers, healthcare professionals may recommend an elimination diet, which consists of systematically removing and reintroducing particular foods. With the assistance of a trained professional, this methodology can assist in ascertaining whether food sensitivities or allergies contribute to the development of tension headaches.

In summary, the implementation of a tension headache-friendly diet necessitates a comprehensive strategy that incorporates consuming well-balanced and consistent meals, ensuring sufficient sleep, engaging in mindful eating, investigating botanical beverages and remedies, and attending to any potential food sensitivities and allergies.

Engaging in deliberate and well-informed decision-making regarding these aspects can substantially contribute to the efficacy of tension headache prevention and management, thereby enhancing overall quality of life and well-being.

CHAPTER FOUR

Alcohol And Tension Headaches: A Moderate Approach To Balance

In addition to alcohol consumption, several lifestyle factors can aggravate tension headaches, which are distinguished by a diffuse, persistent discomfort in the head and neck. A comprehensive comprehension of the correlation between alcohol consumption and tension migraines is imperative for individuals in search of alleviation from this prevalent condition.

Although there is no direct correlation between moderate alcohol consumption and tension migraines, frequent or excessive drinking may contribute to the development or worsening of these symptoms. The dehydration that alcohol is known to induce is a major precipitating factor for tension migraines. It has the potential to cause vasoconstriction, which may impede blood circulation to the brain and give rise to migraines.

Diverse individuals react differently to alcohol, and what one person may perceive as a catalyst may not impact another. Nonetheless, one must exercise prudence regarding personal tolerance and the physiological effects of alcohol. To mitigate the potential discomfort or exacerbation of tension migraines, it is advisable to restrict alcohol consumption and maintain adequate hydration.

A practicable approach would be to select beverages with reduced alcohol content, such as light beer or wine, and to alternate them with water. Additionally, knowing which specific types of alcohol may increase your susceptibility to migraines can assist you in making informed decisions.

Limiting Processed Foods: A Critical Component In The Management Of Tension Headaches

There is evidence linking processed foods, which are frequently loaded with additives, preservatives, and synthetic components, to a range of health complications, such as tension migraines. Limiting one's intake of processed foods may constitute an essential measure in the management and prevention of these migraines.

As catalysts for headaches in susceptible individuals, specific additives, including monosodium glutamate (MSG), nitrates, and artificial sweeteners, have been linked to such effects. In certain studies, MSG, which is frequently present in processed foods and savory treats, has been linked to migraines in particular. Nitrates, which are frequently found in processed meats such as hot dogs and bacon, may also exacerbate headache symptoms in individuals who are overly sensitive to them.

An eating regimen abundant in unprocessed, whole foods—including lean proteins, whole cereals, fruits, and vegetables—can supply vital nutrients while avoiding the headache-inducing substances that may be present in processed foods. This methodology not only promotes holistic well-being but also aids in the regulation of blood glucose levels, thereby diminishing the probability of tension-related migraines.

Engaging in the practice of perusing food labels and exercising discernment when making purchases at the supermarket are fundamental elements of a dietary regimen that aims to reduce the consumption of processed foods. Having greater control over ingredients and preparing meals at home enables one to select fresh, whole foods, which facilitates the avoidance of additives that have the potential to induce tension migraines.

A Holistic Approach To Meal Planning For Tension Headache Prevention

Effective management of tension migraines is significantly aided by meal planning, which encourages a balanced diet and identifies potential triggers. Maintaining proper hydration, establishing regular eating schedules, and integrating nutrient-dense foods are fundamental elements of an efficacious meal strategy designed to avert tension headaches.

Prolonged periods of fasting or skipping meals may result in hypoglycemia, which has the potential to induce tension migraines. Achieving consistent mealtimes and integrating refreshments as necessary can contribute to the regulation of blood sugar levels, thereby diminishing the probability of experiencing migraines.

A diverse range of nutrient-dense foods should be incorporated into one's diet to promote overall health and potentially aid in the prevention of tension headaches. A balanced diet should consist of whole cereals, fruits, vegetables, lean proteins, and healthy fats. There is a possibility that certain foods, such as omega-3 fatty acid-rich salmon or magnesium-rich nuts and legumes, could reduce the prevalence of headaches for some individuals.

It is essential to maintain adequate hydration to prevent tension migraines, as dehydration is a frequent precipitating factor. It is crucial to maintain a sufficient water intake throughout the day and to contemplate the inclusion of hydrating foods, such as fruits and vegetables that are abundant in water, in your meals.

In addition to providing essential nutrients, a comprehensive meal plan fosters a consistent and stable physiological milieu, thereby diminishing the probability of tension migraines. Seeking the advice of a registered dietitian can offer individualized direction in the formulation of a meal regimen customized to one's particular requirements and inclinations.

Engaging In Consultations With Healthcare Professionals: The Significance Of Expert Opinion

Although implementing lifestyle modification and adopting a diet that is conducive to tension headaches may yield positive results, it is imperative to seek the guidance of a healthcare professional to develop a comprehensive strategy for managing headaches. Tailored recommendations can be provided by healthcare professionals, including neurologists and headache specialists, by an individual's medical history, symptoms, and unique triggers.

It is especially critical to seek professional assistance when tension migraines are persistent, severe, or have a substantial negative impact on one's quality of life. By performing a comprehensive assessment, a medical professional can rule out any pre-existing medical conditions and identify potential triggers that are unique to your situation.

Medication management may be advised in certain cases to mitigate the symptoms of tension headaches. Medications may consist of muscle relaxants, analgesics, or preventative measures, contingent upon the frequency and intensity of migraines. It is crucial to establish a close collaboration with your healthcare provider to determine an individualized treatment plan that is both efficacious and tolerable.

Furthermore, healthcare experts possess the ability to offer significant perspectives on lifestyle adjustments, such as dietary modifications, which could potentially supplement medical treatment. Their expertise can assist you in unraveling the intricacies of headache triggers, including the identification of particular foods or environmental elements that might be the source of your tension headaches.

In summary, the management of tension migraines via dictary means necessitates a comprehensive strategy that takes into account factors such as alcohol consumption, ingestion of processed foods, and overall meal preparation. Although it is advantageous to make well-informed dietary decisions, seeking guidance from a healthcare professional guarantees a comprehensive approach that is customized to your specific requirements and situation.

By adopting a healthy lifestyle and seeking professional advice, individuals can strive to effectively manage and prevent tension migraines, thereby enhancing their overall state of health.

Conclusion

In summary, incorporating a meticulously planned dietary regimen into one's regimen may prove to be a beneficial strategy in the management of tension migraines. Although dietary modifications may not entirely eradicate these migraines, they can make a substantial contribution to the alleviation of symptoms and enhancement of overall health. Avoiding potential trigger foods, including those that contain additives, caffeine, and specific preservatives, is crucial. It is imperative to regulate blood sugar levels by consuming balanced meals regularly in order to prevent fluctuations that may contribute to the onset of headaches.

Moreover, sufficient hydration is a critical factor in the prevention of headaches; therefore, it is imperative to give precedence to water consumption throughout the day. The potential benefits of consuming foods abundant in magnesium, which are recognized for their ability to relax muscles, may be enhanced in conjunction with headache relief.

It is imperative to acknowledge that individual reactions to particular foods can differ, thus advocating for the practice of maintaining a food journal and monitoring personal triggers. Furthermore, tailored recommendations can be obtained by seeking the counsel of a registered dietitian or healthcare professional, who can analyze an individual's dietary preferences and medical background.

A tension headache diet is, at its core, a comprehensive strategy that serves as a supplement to additional lifestyle adjustments and medical interventions. By incorporating these dietary strategies into their routines, in conjunction with stress management techniques and suitable medical attention, individuals can improve their capacity to regulate tension migraines and diminish their frequency and severity.

THE END